The Easy Ketogenic Diet Cookbook: 5 Ingredients or Less, Low-Carb, High-Fat Recipes for Weight Loss.

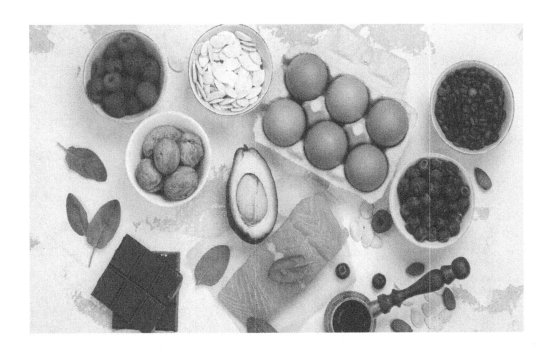

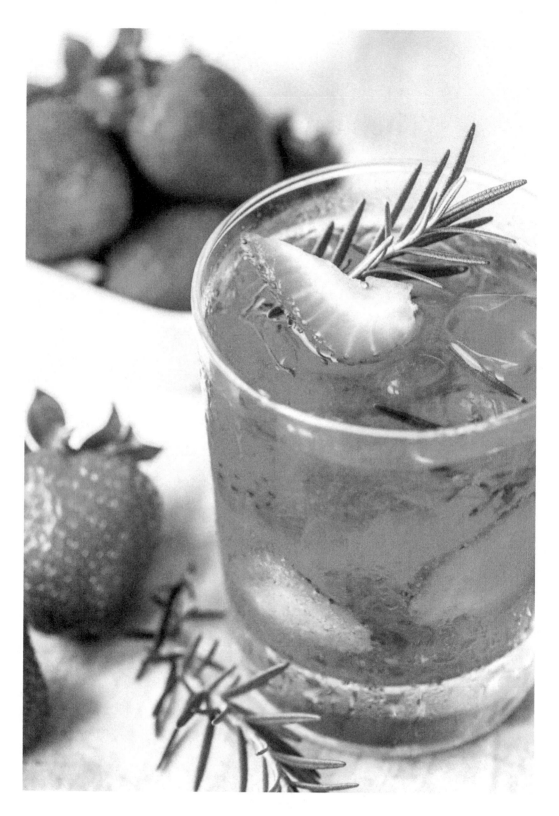

Table of contents:

Introduction _____ *5*

How Does the Keto Diet Work? _____ *7*

Health Benefits of the Ketogenic diet _____ *9*

What Can You Eat? _____ *13*

What to Avoid? _____ *14*

Main Guidelines and Needed Kitchen Equipment _____ *17*

Harmless Weight Loss Tips _____ *22*

Recipes _____ *31*

   Seafood _____ **31**

      Salmon with Zesty Cream Sauce _____ 32

      Crispy Coconut Shrimp _____ 34

      Lemon Baked Cod with Parmesan Cheese_____ 36

      Spicy Tuna Avocado Boats_____ 38

      Cajun Crab Cakes _____ 39

      Asian Glazed Salmon & Cauliflower Rice _____ 41

      Light Shrimp and Bacon Zoodles_____ 43

      Prosciutto Wrapped Scallops and Spinach _____ 45

      Baked Lobster Tails with Garlic Butter _____ 47

      Baked Salmon with Pesto and Tomatoes _____ 49

   Poultry _____ **50**

      Indian Tikka Masala Chicken & Butter_____ 51

      Roasted Chicken with Feta & Olives _____ 53

      Easy Stuffed Chicken _____ 55

      Turkey Meatball & Zoodles _____ 57

      Creamy Chicken Cajun _____ 59

      Chicken Parmesan on a Skillet _____ 61

      Crispy Chicken Tenders_____ 63

      Turkey Breast Nachos_____ 65

      Chicken Club Lettuce Wraps_____ 67

      Tarragon Roasted Chicken_____ 68

   Pork _____ **70**

      Pizza-style Pork Rinds _____ 71

      Easy Spicy Pork Chops _____ 73

      Easy Bacon Wrapped Pork Tenderloin _____ 75

      Sausage, Shrimp and Zucchini Skewers _____ 77

      Low Carb Scotch Eggs_____ 79

Cheese-stuffed Pork Meatballs _____ 80
Low Carb Asian Spare Ribs _____ 82
Sausage Rolls _____ 83
Creamy Marsala Wine Pork _____ 85
Onion and Bacon Smothered Pork Chops _____ 87

Beef _____ **89**
Aromatic Roast Beef _____ 90
Beef Filled Zucchini Boats _____ 92
Red Wine Marinated Beef Skewers _____ 94
Chipotle Spicy Steak _____ 96
Cheeseburger Wraps _____ 97
Cheddar Jalapeno Meatloaf _____ 98
Grilled Steak and Creamy Mushroom Sauce _____ 100
Philly Cheesesteak Stuffed Peppers _____ 102
Beef and Eggs Breakfast Muffins _____ 104
Low Carb Beef Stroganoff _____ 106

Vegetarian _____ **107**
Grilled Halloumi Bruschetta _____ 108
Cheddar Ranch Roasted Cauliflower _____ 109
Wild Mushroom Soup with Crème Fraiche _____ 110
Grilled Vegetable Salad with Olive Oil and Feta _____ 112
Low-Carb Pumpkin and Coconut Cream Soup _____ 114
Keto Avocado Pesto Noodles _____ 116
Roasted Radishes with Soy Sauce _____ 117
Cheesy Vegan Zoodles _____ 119
Cauliflower Mac & Cheese _____ 120
Caprese Grilled Eggplant Roll-ups _____ 122

Drinks and Desserts _____ **124**
Strawberry Coconut Smoothie _____ 125
Keto Avocado Ice Cream _____ 126
Ketto Chai Latte _____ 127
Sugar-free Lemon Curd _____ 128
Keto Peanut Butter Cookies _____ 130

Conclusion _____ *131*

Bonus 14-day Meal Plan _____ **134**
Week 1: _____ **134**
Week 2: _____ **135**

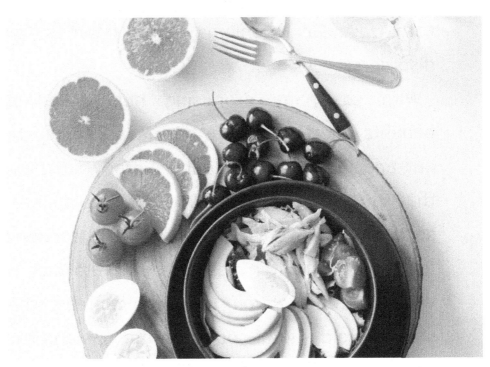

Introduction

The Keto diet has taken the diet, health and fitness world by storm for quite a few reasons - it's easy to follow, doesn't put your system under exhaustion and stress, and produces a wide variety of health benefits including weight loss, cholesterol balance, diabetes control, and blood glucose regulation to name a few. It has even been recognized as a major diet of choice by Mayo Clinic, International Heart Association and other health organizations for treating patients suffering from cardiovascular problems and nervous system disorders.

With so many promising health and fitness benefits, more and more people are trying the diet out and if you haven't done already so, I suggest that you do so, following the guidelines and sections are given in this book. The sections that follow will enlighten you on how Keto diet works, what it can do for you, what you can eat, what you should avoid and of course, some tips and tricks to get you started properly. I know that info regarding Keto diet over the net and books is quite overwhelming and so I have made things clearer and easier to follow, with this book.

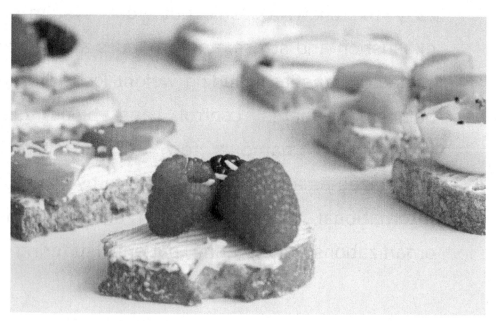

How Does the Keto Diet Work?

The Keto diet is named and based essentially on the concept of "Ketosis". Ketosis is a natural body process, in which the system produces little fat molecules called "ketones". These molecules act as an alternative source of fuel on the body, in place of carbs and sugar, whenever the latter aren't present or are in very short amounts.

When you eat something rich in carbs or sugar, your system will react by producing high amounts of insulin and glucose (blood sugar). Glucose, in this case, is utilized directly by the system to produce short-term energy while insulin is needed to metabolize that glucose and convert it into energy. The problem here is though that the system can only produce temporary spikes in energy as blood glucose isn't sustainable enough to produce energy long-term. And not only this, repeat consumption of carbs and sugar can trigger a series of inflammatory responses within the system which lead to all kinds of problems--from weight gain to diabetes and heart problems.

This is where Ketones can be used as an alternative fuel to energize your system. Ketones are only released by your system through the liver whenever you eat a diet rich in protein and healthy fats and low on carbs and sugar. And contrary to consuming carbs and sugar, when your body is in a ketosis status, the energy preserved is slowly released and more long-lasting and sustainable. Additionally, ketosis fights inflammation and encourages cell regeneration, which is very useful in treating a wide variety of health ailments, as we'll examine below.

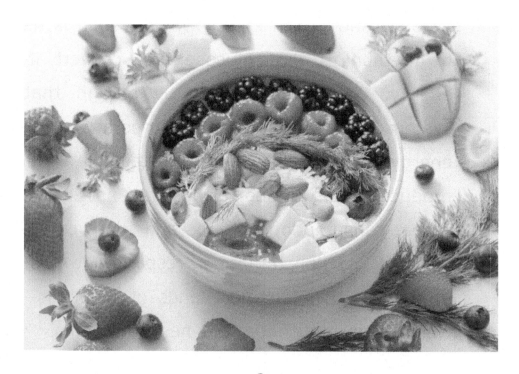

Health Benefits of the Ketogenic diet

Due to the fact that the Ketogenic diet produces Ketones, which are used an alternative and healthier energy source to fuel our systems, a Keto Diet plan yields the following health benefits:

Weight loss. This is among the top 3 most popular uses of Keto diet. Since the body can't take energy from carbs and sugars, the ketosis directs the system to draw energy from stored fat deposits and as you have guessed it, it gets this energy by burning these fat cells first. As your blood glucose and insulin levels drop, your body switches to a fat-burning machine and you can lose fat much easier than opting for a high carb/ low-fat diet, which is the exact opposite of Keto.

Several studies examining the weight loss effects of Keto diet in overweight patients have found that the Keto diet can shrink body fat and lower cholesterol and lipid levels by as much as 40% within 16 weeks/4 months.

Blood Sugar & Diabetes control. Another popular health benefit of Keto diet which makes the diet recommended by many Diabetologists worldwide and doctors whose patients have elevated blood sugar in general. In some studies, it was found that a diet rich in healthy fats like Keto was far more effective in treating blood sugar imbalances as opposed to a simple low-calorie diet. Therefore, if you are in a pre-diabetic status or suffer from Diabetes already, it would be wise to follow a Keto diet to help regulate your blood sugar before it goes out of control.

Cholesterol & Blood Pressure. Keto diet has also been found to help regulate cholesterol and blood lipid levels that are mostly connected to the blockage of arteries by accumulated fat and plaque. More specifically, it has been found that high-fat/low-carb diets like Keto can raise significantly HDL levels (the good cholesterol) while reducing damaging LDL levels (the bad cholesterol). Some studies also show that Keto diets can also help keep blood pressure under control, preventing any extreme drops or raises which can make the person feel ill.

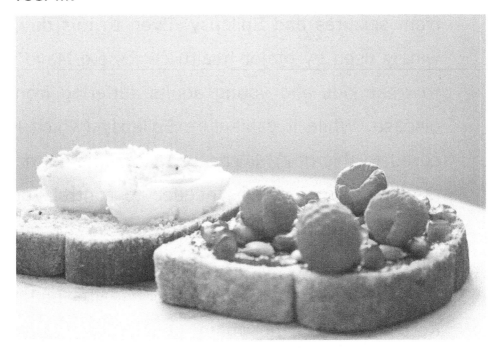

Elevated and Long-lasting Energy Boost. As said in an earlier section, Keto diet acts as an alternative and more sustainable source for producing energy and fueling the system. For this reason, it can be used to boost your energy in periods of stress and pressure e.g working or exams. Unlike munching on a salty and carb snack or sweet, a keto diet food or snack will give you the energy that you'll need to survive through a tough and demanding day without leading to all these infamous energy crashes.

Epilepsy Control. The Keto diet has been utilized for nearly a century to help treat patients suffering from seizures and Epilepsy. Even to this day, it is widely used by major health clinics e.g Mayo Clinic to treat kids and young adults suffering from the disease. While it can't cure Epilepsy (which is not cured to this day), it can certainly help control the number of medications needed to control Epilepsy symptoms and ease inflammation of the nervous system.

Acne and Eczema. Another health benefit of Keto diet, which not many people are aware of, is helping ease acne and eczema breakouts, as well as other inflammatory skin disorders (dermatitis, scalp issues). It is said that the Keto diet can do this by decreasing inflammation inside the body and encouraging tissue cells to repair themselves faster and more effectively than before. It appears to have the opposite effect of following high-carb and high-sugar diets, which have been found to indirectly cause acne and skin inflammation in general.

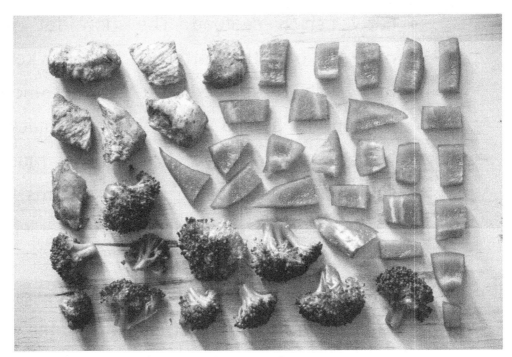

What Can You Eat?

So to cut to the chase, as Keto diet is all about eating certain foods while avoiding others, here a list of all the main foods that should consist 80+% of your daily calorie intake:

- All kinds of unprocessed meat cuts or freshly ground meats e.g beef (steaks, ground beef, chucks, beef liver), pork (cutlets, loin, ham leg, bacon freshly ground pork, pork rinds etc), chicken & poultry (all edible parts), lamb, and whole eggs.

- Fatty fish & seafood. The more fat a fish naturally has, the better for inducing ketosis. Fatty fish & seafood you can eat include: salmon, tuna, sea bass, sardines, mackerel, kippers, cod, cod liver oil, shrimps, mussels, squid, crab, eel, lobster, scallop & clums.
- Leafy greens e.g kale, spinach, lettuce, broccoli, etc.
- Root vegetables e.g carrots, rhubarb, ginger, turnips, taro, celery root, shallots, yams.
- Avocados, olives, and Macadamia.
- High-fat dairy products e.g full-fat greek yogurt, butter (not margarine), heavy cream.
- MTCs fats (coconut oil, wheatgerm oil, cold pressed palm kernel oil)
- Plain water, herbal tea (no sugar added) and vegetable-based juices and smoothies.

What to Avoid?

The following list of foods should not be necessarily avoided completely, but you should aim ideally to consume these in lower amounts and specifically less than 20% of your daily calorie and macro intake.

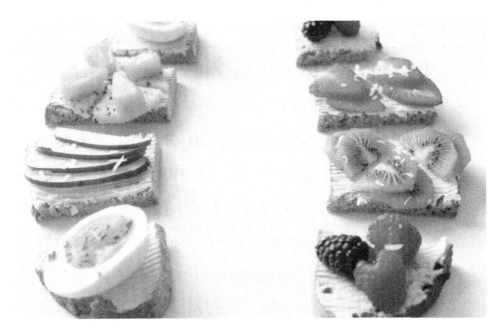

- Processed food that contains carbs and additives e.g canned corned beef, canned tuna, hamburgers, sausage rolls, etc.
- Potatoes and all its by-products e.g crisps, mashed potatoes, potato starch.
- Gluten-based pies, cakes, cookies and sweets
- White rice
- Bread
- Pasta (gluten-free pasta are ok)
- Sugary juices and fizzy drinks

- High glycemic index fruits e.g bananas, pineapples, kiwis, and watermelon
- Beer and alcohol
- Ketchup

In regards to eating nuts and seeds, there are conflicting opinions as to whether they should be included in a Keto diet plan or not, but most agree that you can eat them in moderation and only to supplement other main Keto foods e.g an egg and lettuce salad rather than being consumed as full snacks or meal replacements.

Also regarding oils, it would be wise to use mostly oils that are high in fat and are able to tolerate high heat when cooked or fried. Ghee, coconut oil, palm kernel oil, lard, and tallow are the best for this purpose. Olive oil and safflower oil are also fine in moderation as long as they are not heated enough to oxidize and produce inflammatory molecules.

Note: be careful of processed food and instant meals as they may contain hidden carbs and sugar. Same goes for commercial bought fizzy drinks, energy drinks, and juices or store-bought smoothies. It's best to check the full list of ingredients and if you see more than 4-5 grams of carbs or sugars per 100 ml of product, ditch the product for something more keto-friendly.

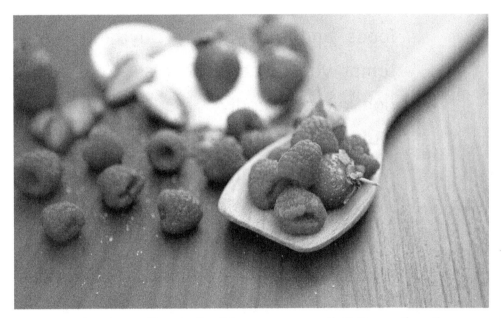

Main Guidelines and Needed Kitchen Equipment

Before we jump onto the recipe section, it would be wise to mention first some kitchen guidelines that will help you to start your Keto diet and stick to it successfully in the long run.

Since our cooking and eating environment does affect our dietary choices, it would be wise to make your surroundings suitable for following a Keto diet, especially if you are switching from a different former diet. Here are some tips:

- Fill your fridge and cabinet with keto-friendly foods and throw away anything that would tempt you to eat otherwise. You can replace non-keto friendly foods with ketogenic alternatives. Remember that foods rich in carbs and sugar are enough to ruin your Ketogenic efforts in an instant--and make you feel like crap afterwards.
- Plan your meals in advance. Since most of us are busy during the weekdays due to work and family obligations, it would be smarter to prepare your week's keto meals in advance at a day or time you will be free. As you can see on the rest of this e-book, the recipes don't take much ingredients and time and so you can spare 2-3 hours on a day that's convenient for you to make them. In case you are traveling, make sure that you have in your bag some quick keto-friendly snacks or

research through your smartphone any keto-friendly restaurants, cafes or menu items near you.

- Stay away from eating an excessive amount of "quickies" and convenient foods. Yes, even some keto-friendly foods e.g high-fat ice cream with stevia can be bad for you if you consume too much of it, because it's convenient for you. It's best for this reason to make one or two servings of these foods that you may be tempted to binge on. If it's out of sight, it's out of your mind as well!

- Only consume foods that you can count and try to stick to your macro targets. Even a little oil, cheese, or extra fat here and there is enough to add up and contribute to weight gain as opposed to weight loss.

Generally speaking, you won't need any fancy and expensive kitchen equipment when on Keto however you will need to expand your kitchen tools and equipment beyond the essentials so you are able to prepare healthy Keto meals easier and faster. Here is what you'll need as a start:

- **Food processor.** A food processor is useful for preparing many different keto-foods like for example cauliflower rice, shredded cheese, and finely chopped veggies without making them totally mashed, as in the case of mixing them in a blender.

- **Immersion hand blender.** This inexpensive mixer is very handy for blending keto soups and making your own whipped cream or even mayo and cold cream sauces.

- **Vegetable spiralizer.** These veggie spiralizers are pretty popular these days as they can make noodles out of almost any long vegetable in seconds. Since most ordinary pasta kinds contain carbs and gluten, you will need a spiralizer to make your own low carb and gluten-free veggie noodles in an instant.

- **Kitchen shears.** These are useful for a wide variety of purposes--from cutting soft vegetables to cutting bacon and deboning meat and chicken thighs easily and fast.

- **Measuring cups.** Since it is important to follow your recipes to a T and count your macros, you will need some ml/gram and cup measuring containers. 2-3 sizes and cup kinds e.g one for liquids and one for dry ingredients are essential.

- **Barbeque or grilling pan.** Nothing beats the taste and joyful experience of having a barbeque in your yard and preparing high-protein and high-fat meals e.g beef brisket or bacon but you can sort of replicate the texture (and taste) for less by using a grilling pan and liquid smoke in your food.

Other optional tools and equipment that will help add more variety to your keto diet are: sous-vide machines, a slow-cooker, muffin tins (for delicious egg-based breakfast muffins), mini whisks, an avocado slicer, and a fondue cheese-making machine if you frequently host parties or invite your friends or family around.

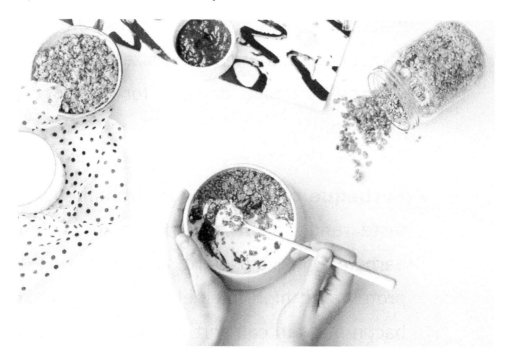

Harmless Weight Loss Tips

With obesity being so widespread in the world that it currently affects 2 in 5 adults, diet options like Keto could be the answer to the worldwide obesity epidemic. Our genetics, environment, and of course diet and lifestyle choices all contribute to this phenomenon. People are prone to eating fattening and unhealthy foods as a result of stress, convenience, and because their friends or family eat so. It's time to unbreak this obesity pattern by implementing more suitable and healthy diets and making healthy lifestyle picks.

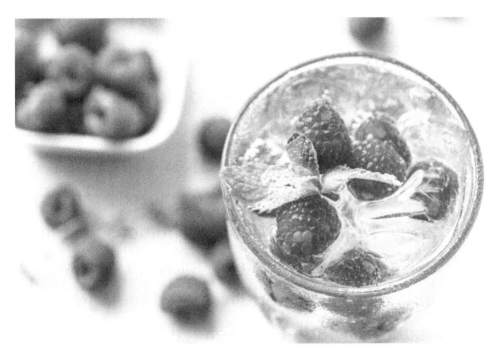

But how can Keto helps us lose weight over other diets? Even though there is much controversy surrounding the topic, new studies have found that it's not only calories that matter when we want to lose weight, either short-term or long-term. Our macro ratios e.g amount of carbs, protein, fats and sugars we consume daily also matters. A recent meta-study conducted by Drs. Kevin Hall, and Juen Guo has revealed very convincing data that regarding the efficient of Keto diet over a low-fat diet. It was found specifically that participants following a Keto diet for several months lost more weight (around 8.8 pounds) on average as opposed to those following low-fat diets. And following a Keto diet also comes with additionally health benefits like cholesterol and blood sugar control.

However, despite the above findings, the Ketogenic diet for weight loss can trigger a series of short-term yet unpleasant side effects. Also, people with certain health conditions should consult their doctors first before going on Keto as ketones can crash with certain medicine ingredients and produce unwanted side effects.

In some cases, new Keto diet beginners may experience flu-like symptoms for a few days to a week or two as they switch from their old diet to Keto. People with problems like hypothyroidism, adrenal fatigue, and hormonal balances will have the most trouble adjusting to a Keto diet.

In the case of hypercholesterolemia sufferers, a high-fat diet would be hard as they lack the necessary genes to receive and process the LDL (good fat) compound properly. This is why doctors advise such patients to follow a high protein and fiber and low-fat/low-carb diet as opposed to Keto.

Also, those affected by hypothyroidism and adrenal fatigue will struggle a bit more to adjust to the Keto diet as a result of insulin, blood glucose, and hormonal implications. When insulin levels drop, the switch of the inactive T-4 hormone compound to the T-3 is hindered, which can trigger the onset of thyroid issues. The adrenals react by releasing epinephrine, cortisol, and norepinephrine to serve as pseudo-hormones which are necessary for several body functions e.g heart palpitation and energy release. Additionally, the fall of T-3 hormone levels can also lead to an unhealthy spike of cholesterol levels. Therefore, if you are begging a Keto diet when you have these issues, restricting carbs make matters worse.

To avoid or at least control any health implications as a result of starting your Keto diet when you have hormonal balance issues, it is important that you take enough of your calories from nutrient-rich foods, protein and healthy fats (in a lesser degree). These will be enough to fuel your system so it can waste its glycogen, help recover thyroid function, and save you from trouble.

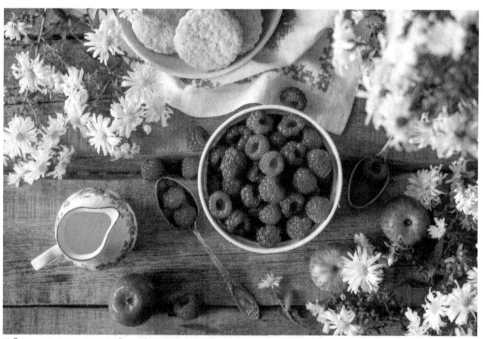

If you are feeling a bit tired and sluggish after eating a meal that is high in fat, but very low (or zero) in carbs, you can eat a small dose of healthy carbs like lima beans, sweet potatoes, or nuts and seeds so that your energy is restored back to normal. The macro ratio of fats and protein to carbs should be a bit different to suit your case and preferably 60-70% proteins and fats and 30% carbs as opposed to 80% fats, protein and fiber and 20% or fewer carbs.

Now, there are other types of People who also have specific dietary requirements and these are pregnant and breastfeeding women, and those who had gallbladder removal surgery.

Those who had a gallbladder removal surgery may have to consider the following:

- Control and measure the level of fat you take daily as a start and increase gradually over two weeks.
- Take an ox bile or lipase supplement with every meal.
- Avoid consuming too much fat in one serving without any other macros e.g protein and fiber.

Pregnant or breastfeeding women may also have to take into account the following tips when switching to a Keto diet:

- Eat foods abundance of micronutrients. It is important during your pregnancy to eat plenty of micronutrients that will support you and the baby during pregnancy and breastfeeding and that going on Keto, doesn't mean that you should refrain from eating nutrient-rich foods, as long as they aren't high on carbs or sugars. Micronutrients for pregnancy include folic acid, magnesium, Vitamin E, Iron, iodine and Omega-3 fatty acids. Some good keto-friendly and nutrient dense foods are beef steaks and liver, beef stock, dark leafy greens, dried seaweed and fatty fish.
- Raise your protein consumption during the first few months of pregnancy. As protein is an essential building block of muscle and tissue in general and your macro requirements during pregnancy are higher, you should aim to consume at least 1 and 1.2 grams/pound of lean mass during this period.

- Gradually raise your barb intake during the last stages of pregnancy and breastfeeding. During the last 2 months of pregnancy to labor and finally breastfeeding, you can add an additional 50 grams of extra carbs e.g rice or pasta, and fruits like bananas to help you produce more milk.

Tip: Consult your doctor before trying a Keto diet when breastfeeding as it may lead to unwanted side effects.

Keep in mind that as each of us has a different system and reacts differently to foods, food combos and diet plans in general, and so it would be wise to experiment a little with foods and recipes that make you feel your best and make you lose weight (along with other health benefits). It's natural to feel a bit unwell once you switch to Keto, but if symptoms persist for more than 1-2 weeks or are totally unbearable, you should either try to switch your macronutrient ratios and eat a tad more carbs or stop and switch back to your normal diet. However, in most cases with no serious health issues, side effects are minimal and only last a few days to a week.

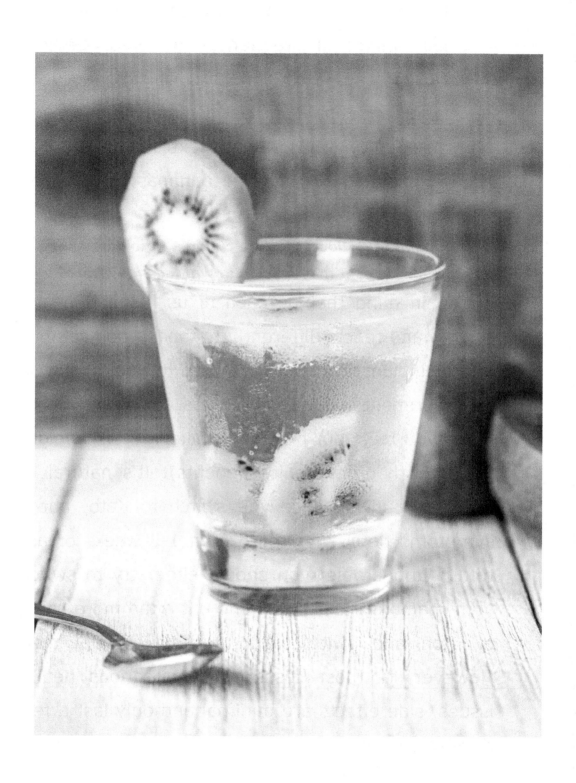

Recipes

Seafood

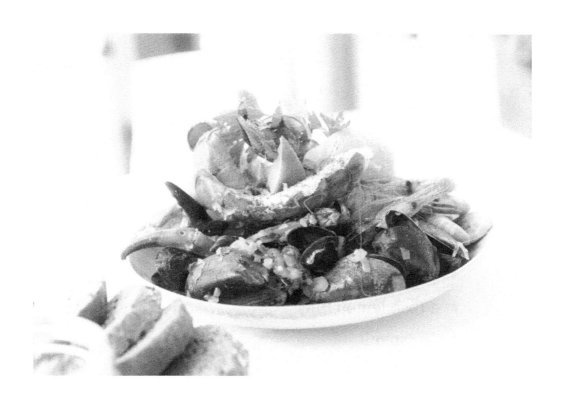

Salmon with Zesty Cream Sauce

Servings: 2

Cooking time: 10 minutes

Prep time: 5-7 minutes

Nutritional Info (per serving):

Calories: 397

Fat: 22.7

Carbs: 4.2 g

Protein: 42.0 g

Ingredients:

- 2 boneless salmon or trout fillets
- ⅓ cup sour cream
- 2 tsp mustard
- 1 tbsp lemon juice
- ½ tsp dill
- 1 tsp lemon zest

Directions:

- Mix all the cream ingredients and spices together in a small bowl.
- Season with salt and pepper to taste and set aside.

- Lightly grease a shallow pan and cook the fillets for 2-3 minutes on each side (for a medium to well-done result).
- Serve on a dish and pour the sauce on top or on the side. You can serve it also with some broccoli or asparagus for an extra kick of taste and nutrients.

Crispy Coconut Shrimp

Servings: 4 servings

Cooking time: 20 minutes

Prep time: 5 minutes

Nutritional Info (per serving):

Calories: 354

Fat: 24 g

Carbs: 20 g

Protein: 13 g

Ingredients:

- 1 pound of large shrimp (peeled and deveined)
- ⅓ cup coconut flour
- 1 tsp cayenne seasoning (salt included)
- 3 eggs beaten
- ½ cup unsweetened coconut flakes

Directions:

- Keep the coconut flour with the seasoning, coconut flakes, and beaten eggs into separate bowls each.
- Dip and roll in the shrimps (one by one) into the coconut flour mixture, shake of the excess flour, dip

in the eggs and then roll in last to the unsweetened coconut flakes.

- Heat one cup of oil and dry the shrimps for 4-5 minutes or until golden brown.

- Serve in a shallow dish with absorbing paper and serve with hot mayo (mayo with cayenne seasoning).

Lemon Baked Cod with Parmesan Cheese

Servings: 3

Cooking time: 15 minutes

Prep time: 15 minutes

Nutritional Info (per serving):

Calories: 410

Fat: 20 g

Protein: 49 g

Carbs: 3 g

Ingredients:

- 1 ½ pounds of cod fillets
- ¾ cup grated parmesan cheese
- 1 lemon, juiced (zest kept separate)
- 1 tbsp fresh parsley, chopped
- 4 tbsp salted butter, melted

Directions:

- Preheat the oven to 400F/200C.
- Pad the cod fillets with paper to remove excess moisture.
- Place the melted butter into a shallow bowl.

- In a separate bowl, combine the parmesan cheese and parsley together.
- Dip each of the fish fillets first into the butter and then to parmesan cheese and parsley mixture so you form a light crust.
- Bake the crusted fillets in a baking dish in the oven for 15-18 minutes.
- Add a bit of lemon juice on top and serve.

Spicy Tuna Avocado Boats

Servings: 2

Cooking time: 0

Prep time: 3 minutes

Nutritional Info (per serving):

Calories: 256

Fat: 17.84

Protein: 15 g

Carbs: 7.31 g

Ingredients:

- 2 avocados halved
- ½ lb of sushi grade ahi tuna (or smoked tuna if you can't find any)
- 2 tbsp of mayo
- 1-2 sriracha sauce
- 1 tsp of toasted sesame seeds

Directions:

- Combine in a small bowl the tuna, with the mayo, sriracha sauce and toasted sesame seeds.
- Scoop and distribute the mixture onto the avocado halves.
- Add optionally some extra sriracha sauce on top.

Cajun Crab Cakes

Servings: 4-5

Cooking time: 7-8 min

Prep time: 5 min

Nutritional Info (per serving):

Calories: 320

Fat: 22 g

Protein: 25 g

Carbs: 3 g

Ingredients:

- 1 lb crab meat, shredded
- ⅓ cup flaxseed meal
- 1 tsp of salted cajun seasoning
- 2 eggs
- 1 tbsp of Worcestershire sauce

Directions:

- Combine all the dry ingredients in a bowl
- Add the crab meat and mix in the eggs and Worcestershire sauce until well combined. You should end up with a semi-mushy texture that you

can easily scoop and make into a patty. If the mixture is too thick/dry, add a more Worcestershire sauce,

- Form the mixture into patties and shallow fry in a lightly greased pan for 3 minutes on each side.
- Serve hot and ideally with Cajun mayo.

Asian Glazed Salmon & Cauliflower Rice

Servings: 4

Cooking time: 10 min

Prep time: 5 min

Nutritional Info (per serving):

Calories: 210

Fat: 13 g

Protein: 15.38 g

Carbs: 4 g

Ingredients:

- 4 boneless fillets of salmon
- 2 cups (around 550 grams) of frozen cauliflower rice (or freshly ground cauliflower rice using a food processor)
- 4 tbsp of liquid aminos or soy sauce
- 2 tbsp of shallots, chopped finely
- 2 tbsp of sesame oil

Directions:

- Make a marinade of the liquid aminos, shallots, and sesame oil and combine them all into a bowl.

- Soak the salmon fillets to the marinade and optionally refrigerate for at least an hour before cooking.
- Pop these into the oven and bake for 10-12 minutes.
- While the salmon cooks, heat and prepare the frozen cauliflower rice, according to package instructions.
- Serve the salmon over the cauliflower rice hot.

Light Shrimp and Bacon Zoodles

Servings: 4

Cooking time: 12 min

Prep time: 2 min

Nutritional Info (per serving):

Calories: 698

Fat: 51 g

Protein: 48 g

Carbs: 6 g

Ingredients:

- 1 lb of fresh peeled and deveined shrimp
- ¼ cup of salted butter
- 2 cloves of garlic mashed
- 2-3 stripes of bacon, chopped
- 1 zucchini, made into zoodles using a spiralizer or mandolin slicer

Directions:

- Heat a skillet, add the butter and shrimp and cook for 2 minutes on each side.
- Add the garlic and cook for another minute.

- Remove the shrimps from the heat and add the bacon and the zucchini noodles in the garlic oil. Cook tossing for 4-5 minutes.
- Return the shrimps to the bacon zoodles, toss, and transfer to a deep dish.
- Sprinkle optionally with some freshly grated parmesan.

Prosciutto Wrapped Scallops and Spinach

Servings: 4

Cooking time: 15 min

Prep time: 5 min

Nutritional Info (per serving):

Calories: 214

Fat: 13 g

Protein: 18 g

Carbs: 6 g

Ingredients:

- 12 large dry scallops
- 3 slices of prosciutto, cut into 12 thin strips (to wrap the scallops)
- ½ tsp of lemon pepper
- 12 oz. of fresh baby spinach
- 3 tbsp of olive oil

Directions:

- Wrap the scallops each with a slice of prosciutto and secure with a toothpick. Season with lemon pepper.
- Place on a baking sheet and bake for 6-8 minutes on the broiler of the oven.

- As the scallops cook, add a spinach with the olive oil and some extra lemon pepper on top to cook until wilted for 3-4 minutes on high hear. Reserve.
- Take 3 scallops for each serving and arrange the cooked spinach on the sides and serve.

Baked Lobster Tails with Garlic Butter

Servings: 2

Cooking time: 15 min

Prep time: 5 min

Nutritional Info (per serving):

Calories: 222

Fat: 14 g

Protein: 21 g

Carbs: 2 g

Ingredients:

- 4 lobster tails
- 1 lemon juiced
- 5 cloves of garlic
- ¼ cup grated parmesan
- 4 tbsp of salted butter

Directions:

- Preheat oven to 375F/180C. In a small bowl combine together the lemon juice, garlic, and grated parmesan.

- Using kitchen shears cut the clear skin and remove off the lobster and brush the tails with the garlic butter mix.
- Place on a baking sheet with parchment paper on top and bake in the oven for 15 minutes.

Baked Salmon with Pesto and Tomatoes

Servings: 2

Cooking time: 15 min

Prep time: 10 min

Nutritional Info (per serving):

Calories: 364

Fat: 18.6 g

Protein: 43.1 g

Carbs: 3.6 g

Ingredients:

- 2 wild Alaskan boneless salmon fillets
- 2 tbsp of basic pesto
- 1 large tomato, chopped
- 2 tbsp of olive oil
- Salt

Directions:

- Season the salmon fillets with salt.
- Arrange in baking dish, wrap with olive oil and add 1 tbsp of pesto on top of each salmon.
- Add 2 tomato slices over the salmon and pesto.
- Bake for 15 minutes. Serve with an arugula salad or cauliflower rice.

Poultry

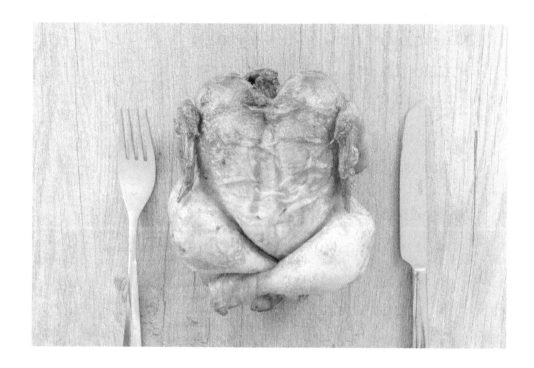

Indian Tikka Masala Chicken & Butter

Servings: 3-4

Cooking time: 15 min

Prep time: 5 min

Nutritional Info (per serving):

Calories: 880

Fat: 87.4 g

Protein: 24.8 g

Carbs: 13 g

Ingredients:

- 3 boneless chicken thighs, sliced
- 75 grams/or ½ cup Tikka Masala Paste
- 1 cup of coconut cream
- 2 tbsp of butter or ghee
- 1 tbsp of garlic salt

Directions:

- In a small bowl, combine the paste with the coconut cream.
- Season the chicken thighs with garlic salt, heat the butter and add to the skillet. Cook the thighs for 4-5 minutes.

- Add the tikka masala paste and coconut cream mixture, stir to cover the chicken thighs and cook for another minute.
- Serve on deep dish or bowl over a bed of basmati rice.

Roasted Chicken with Feta & Olives

Servings: 4

Cooking time: 50 min

Prep time: 5 min

Nutritional Info (per serving):

Calories: 574

Fat: 34 g

Protein: 32 g

Carbs: 8 g

Ingredients:

- 1 half chicken, cut into pieces
- 3 tbsp of olive oil
- ⅓ cup feta, crumbled
- 1/2 cup of black, pitted olives
- Salt/Pepper

Directions:

- Preheat the oven to 400F/200C.
- Season the chicken pieces with salt and pepper.
- Place on a baking sheet with the olive oil drizzled on top.

- Cook for 1 hour (40 minutes on the fan and last 10 minutes on the broiler). During the last ten minutes of broiling, add the crumbled feta and kalamata olives.
- Serve with spinach salad or rice.

Easy Stuffed Chicken

Servings: 5

Cooking time: 30 min

Prep time: 10 min

Nutritional Info (per serving):

Calories: 357

Fat: 19.3g

Protein: 42.5 g

Carbs: 1.7 g

Ingredients:

- 4 chicken breasts, skinned and pounded
- 2/3 cup of almond flour
- 3 small eggs, beaten
- 4 slices of cheddar cheese
- 4 slices of ham

Directions:

- Season the chicken breasts with salt and pepper.
- Keep eggs and almond flour into separate shallow bowls each.

- Place a cheese slice and ham slices over each chicken breast. Wrap and roll from edge to edge and secure with a toothpick.
- Dip the stuffed chicken rolls first into the eggs and then the almond flour.

Turkey Meatball & Zoodles

Servings: 2

Cooking time: 12 min

Prep time: 5 min

Nutritional Info (per serving):

Calories: 439

Fat: 20.7 g

Protein: 17 g

Carbs: 8 g

Ingredients:

- 1 pounds ground turkey
- 2-3 shallots, finely chopped
- 2 eggs beaten
- 1 cup of low sugar tomato sauce
- 2 medium zucchinis made into zoodles.

Directions:

- Reserve ⅓ cup of the tomato sauce.
- In a bowl, combine the ground turkey with the reserved ⅓ of tomato sauce, the eggs and the shallots, form into small bowls the size of a golf ball.

- In a preheated oven, place the turkey balls in a shallow baking dish lined with parchment paper and cook for 15 minutes at 380F/200C.
- In a greased pan, add the zoodles, stir and cook for 2-3 minutes until softened a bit and add the tomato sauce. Cook for another 2-3 minutes.
- Serve the meatballs ideally over the cooked zoodles and tomato sauce.

Creamy Chicken Cajun

Servings: 3 servings

Cooking time: 15 min

Prep time: 5 min

Nutritional Info (per serving):

Calories: 450

Fat: 39 g

Protein: 17.4 g

Carbs: 8 g

Ingredients:

- 4 boneless chicken thighs, skin on
- 1 tbsp of cajun seasoning mix
- 1 tbsp of garlic salt
- ½ cup heavy cream
- 1 full tbsp of butter or ghee

Directions:

- Cut the chicken thighs into thick slices and season with the Cajun seasoning mix, making sure that it covers all the pieces evenly.

- Melt the butter on a skillet and add the chicken thighs. Shallow fry for 3 minutes on each side. (They should look white and opaque but still be juicy).
- Add the heavy cream, toss and cook for a minute or so before turning off the heat.
- Serve with cauliflower rice.

Chicken Parmesan on a Skillet

Servings: 4

Cooking time: 15 min

Prep time: 10 min

Nutritional Info (per serving):

Calories: 330

Fat: 17 g

Protein: 37 g

Carbs: 7 g

Ingredients:

- 3-4 large skinless chicken breast halves
- ½ cup of parmesan cheese, grated
- 6 oz. of mozzarella cheese, grated
- 1 tbsp of Italian seasoning mix
- 2 cups of marinara or Italian pasta sauce

Directions:

- Heat a bit of olive oil in a deep skillet (around 3 inches high) and add the chicken breast halves. Season with the Italian seasoning mix and cook for 7-8 minutes (around 4 minutes on each chicken breast side)

- Add the marina sauce and let cook for another 5 minutes, till its gets slightly thickened.
- Add the grated cheeses on top and finish of the dish in the oven (375F/180C) for 8-10 minutes or until the cheese is melted.

Crispy Chicken Tenders

Servings:4

Cooking time: 20 min

Prep time: 10 min

Nutritional Info (per serving):

Calories: 580

Fat: 32 g

Protein: 63 g

Carbs: 4 g

Ingredients:

- 1 lb or 4 pieces of chicken breast
- ¾ flaxseed flour
- 3 eggs beaten
- 1 tbsp of parmesan cheese
- 1 tbsp of garlic salt

Directions:

- In a bowl, combine the flaxseed flour and parmesan cheese with the garlic salt and set aside.
- In another bowl, beat two eggs.
- Cut the chicken breasts into two thick stripes or bite-sized squares.

- Dip each chicken piece first into the egg and then to the dry mixture, making sure that everything is coated evenly.

- Grease a skillet with a bit of oil or butter and shallow dry for 3-4 minutes on each side until golden brown.

- Remove from the heat and serve on a dish with paper and a small bowl of marinara sauce.

Turkey Breast Nachos

Servings: 4

Cooking time: 5 min

Prep time: 5 min

Nutritional Info (per serving):

Calories: 176 g

Fat: 7 g

Protein: 15 g

Carbs: 4 g

Ingredients:

- 4 small to medium size low carb tortillas
- ⅔ cup leftover shredded turkey or chicken roast
- ½ cup of cheddar cheese
- 2 tbsp of salsa
- 1 tbsp of guacamole(optional)

Directions:

- Cut the tortillas into 6-8 triangles (the same way you would cut a pizza).
- Bake in the broiler for around 10 minutes (until they are crisp enough but do not break apart).

- Add to a shallow serving dish and add the shredded turkey on top and the cheddar cheese.
- Pop back into the oven and bake for 7-8 minutes at 380F/200C until cheese is melted.
- Serve optionally with salsa or guacamole.

Chicken Club Lettuce Wraps

Servings: 2

Cooking time: 0

Prep time: 10 min

Nutritional Info (per serving):

Calories: 806

Fat: 70 g

Protein: 38 g

Carbs: 4 g

Ingredients:

- 9 oz. of cooked chicken bites (roasted or boiled)
- 4 slices of fried bacon, chopped
- ½ cup of mayonnaise
- 4 large romaine lettuce leaves
- 1 large tomato seeded and cubed

Directions:

- Combine all the ingredients together except the lettuce leaves in a bowl.
- Distribute the mixture into each lettuce leaf, as if you are filling a boat and serve.

Tarragon Roasted Chicken

Servings: 2

Cooking time: 45 min

Prep time:5 min

Nutritional Info (per serving):

Calories: 461

Fat: 30 g

Protein: 38 g

Carbs: 4 g

Ingredients:

- 2 bone-in chicken thighs
- 2 tbsp of fresh tarragon leaves, chopped
- 2-3 shallots, thoroughly chopped
- 1 tbsp of garlic salt
- 2 tbsp of olive oil

Directions:

- Preheat the oven to 380F/180 C.
- In a small bowl combine the olive oil, garlic salt, and the tarragon with the shallots.
- Brush the mixture over the chicken pieces.

- Bake in a greased baking dish for 40 minutes and switch on the broiler on the last five minutes to form a light crust.
- Serve with salad or cauliflower rice.

Pork

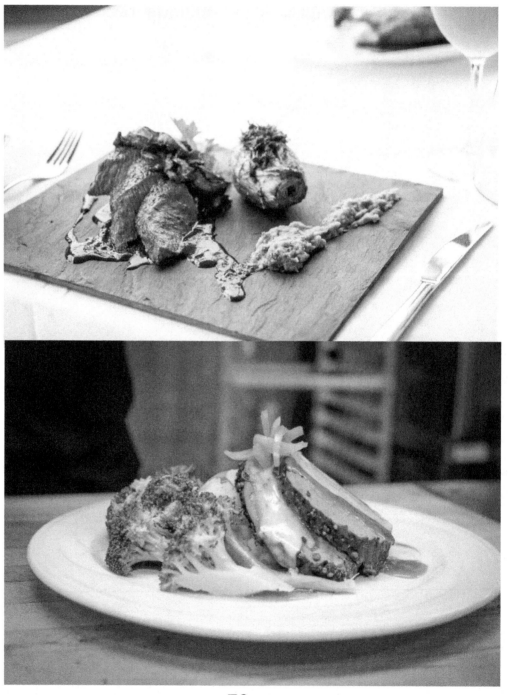

Pizza-style Pork Rinds

Servings: 4

Cooking time: 5 min

Prep time: 5 min

Nutritional Info (per serving):

Calories: 286

Fat: 22 g

Protein:18 g

Carbs: 3.5 g

Ingredients:

- 4 oz of pork rinds
- 2 tbsp of pasta tomato sauce
- 2 tsp of Italian seasoning
- 4 tbsp of salted butter
- 2 tbsp of parmesan cheese or cheese powder

Directions:

- Preheat the oven to 380F/18C.
- In a small bowl, combine the tomato sauce with the butter, the Italian seasoning mix, and the cheese powder.

- Place the pork rinds into a bowl and top with the tomato mixture. Toss well to cover the pork rinds evenly.
- Line everything into a baking dish lined with parchment paper and roast for 7-8 minutes.
- Serve optionally with salad.

Easy Spicy Pork Chops

Servings: 4

Cooking time: 10 min

Prep time: 5 min

Nutritional Info (per serving):

Calories: 277

Fat: 16 g

Protein: 29 g

Carbs: 3 g

Ingredients:

- 4 boneless pork chops
- 1 tbsp of Worcestershire sauce
- 1 tbsp of mixed spice rub for meats
- 1 tsp of onion powder
- 1 tbsp of garlic salt

Directions:

- In large zip bag combine everything except the pork chops. Squish and shake till everything looks combined well.

- Add the pork chops in the bag, close and shake once again so that they are evenly covered with the mixture.
- Cook in a greased grilling pan for 10 minutes (5 minutes on each side).
- Serve ideally with coleslaw salad.

Easy Bacon Wrapped Pork Tenderloin

Servings: 5-6

Cooking time: 30 min

Prep time: 5 min

Nutritional Info (per serving):

Calories: 455

Fat: 25 g

Protein: 52 g

Carbs: 0.8 g

Ingredients:

- 1 lb of pork tenderloin, excess fat removed
- 1 tsp of garlic paste
- 2 tbsp of dry white wine
- 2 tbsp of soy sauce
- 4 slices of bacon

Directions:

- Place the tenderloin in a big plastic bag and add the garlic paste, onion, powder, whine and soy sauce. Shake well and let marinate on the fridge for at least a couple of hours before cooking.

- Transfer the marinated tenderloin onto a cutting board and reserve the marinade aside.
- Line the 4 pieces of bacon next to each other, place the tenderloin on one of the edges and wrap the bacon around it.
- Bake in a preheated oven (380F/180C) for 30 minutes.
- Warm up the marinade in a small pan, add a few drizzles of extra wine or water and once it has started to bubble remove from the heat.
- Pour over the cooked tenderloin and serve ideally with arugula salad.

Sausage, Shrimp and Zucchini Skewers

Servings: 8

Cooking time: 10 min

Prep time: 20 min

Nutritional Info (per serving):

Calories: 178

Fat: 12 g

Protein: 12 g

Carbs: 3 g

Ingredients:

- 3 large smoked sausages cut into 30-35 slices in total
- 2 medium-sized zucchinis, cut into 35-40 slices
- 40 shrimps, peeled with tail on
- 1 batch of low carb barbeque sauce

Directions:

- Take 20 medium skewers and soak in water first so they don't get burned while cooking.
- Take each skewer and thread 2 pieces of shrimp, two of zucchini and two of sausages (one ingredient, then another to make a pattern).

- Brush the barbeque sauce over the shrimp and zucchini and cook over a grill pan for 3-4 minutes on each side.
- Serve optionally with chopped lettuce and some extra barbeque sauce.

Low Carb Scotch Eggs

Servings: 6

Cooking time: 30 min

Prep time: 10 min

Nutritional Info (per serving):

Calories: 352

Fat: 29 g

Protein: 19 g

Carbs: 2 g

Ingredients:

- 6 hard-boiled eggs, peeled
- 1 lb of ground pork sausage meat
- ¼ cup of almond flour
- 1 tbsp of olive oil
- Black pepper

Directions:

- Combine everything in a small bowl except the eggs until you end up with a workable mince-like paste.
- Wrap the mixture around the eggs, making sure that there are no gaps and holes.
- Place on a lightly greased baking dish and cook at 375 F/180C for 12-15 minutes and serve with mayo.

Cheese-stuffed Pork Meatballs

Servings: 6

Cooking time: 20 min

Prep time: 10 min

Nutritional Info (per serving):

Calories: 445

Fat: 32 g

Protein: 30 g

Carbs: 1 g

Ingredients:

- 10 oz of ground pork
- 20 oz of ground pork sausage
- 2 eggs
- 3 large cheese strings
- 1 tbsp of Italian seasoning

Directions:

- Preheat the oven to 380F/180C.
- Combine all the ingredients together in a bowl except the cheese strings
- Cut the cheese strings into several small pieces (around 22-24 in number)

- Take a mini handful of the pork mixture and place a cheese piece inside then cover with extra pork mixture and roll into a bowl (the cheese should appear concealed).
- Bake in a greased baking dish for 20 minutes.
- Serve with salad and tomato sauce.

Low Carb Asian Spare Ribs

Servings: 7-8

Cooking time: 80 min

Prep time: 5 min

Nutritional Info (per serving):

Calories: 312

Fat: 9.2 g

Protein: 37.2 g

Carbs: 12 g

Ingredients:

- 3 lbs (around two average racks) of pork spare ribs
- 1 medium shallot, chopped
- ½ cup of soy sauce
- 1 clove of garlic
- 1 tsp of crushed anise seeds

Directions:

- Combine all the ingredients except the spare ribs to make a marinade in a small bowl.
- Make small incisions between the ribs (do not cut fully) and brush the soy sauce mixture onto the spare rib racks.
- Cook in preheated oven for 1 ½ hour before serving.

Sausage Rolls

Servings: 4-5

Cooking time: 20 min

Prep time: 20 min

Nutritional Info (per serving):

Calories: 583

Fat: 47 g

Protein: 34 g

Carbs: 7 gr

Ingredients:

- 1 lb of raw, ground pork sausage meat
- 2 tbsp cream cheese
- ⅔ cups almond flour
- ½ cup shredded mozzarella
- 1 egg beaten

Directions:

- Preheat the oven to 380F/180C.
- Mix together the cream cheese, the almond flour, the mozzarella, and the beaten egg in a bowl to make a dough.

- Roll the dough into a large rectangle with roller dusted with some almond flour. Cut in half.
- Divide the pork sausage meat over the middle the two cut dough pieces, leaving around ½ inch blank on the sides.
- Roll the dough from one side of the dough to the other, lengthwise. Repeat the same with the other dough piece.
- Turn it over and cut into 8 pieces each.
- Place on a baking dish with lined parchment paper.
- Bake in the oven for around 15-18 minutes before serving.

Creamy Marsala Wine Pork

Servings: 4

Cooking time: 15 min

Prep time: 5 min

Nutritional Info (per serving):

Calories: 260

Fat: 13 g

Protein: 25 g

Carbs: 4 g

Ingredients:

- 1 lb. pork tenderloin, sliced and lightly pounded
- ½ cup of white mushrooms chopped
- ⅓ cup of marsala red wine
- ⅓ cup of heavy cream
- 2 tbsp of salted butter

Directions:

- Heat a pan with the butter and add the pork tenderloins.
- Cook for 3-4 minutes on each side until golden brown but not dry.

- Add the mushrooms and saute for another couple of minutes.
- Add the wine, increase the heat and let in till it evaporates.
- Finish off with the heavy cream, toss for an extra 1-2 minutes and remove from the heat.
- Serve with salad or cauliflower rice.

Onion and Bacon Smothered Pork Chops

Servings: 4

Cooking time: 40 min

Prep time: 10 min

Nutritional Info (per serving):

Calories: 352

Fat: 18.2 g

Protein: 37 g

Carbs: 4 g

Ingredients:

- 4 bone-in pork chops
- 5 slices of bacon, chopped
- 1 small onion, sliced
- ¼ cup heavy cream
- Salt/Pepper

Directions:

- In a skillet, throw in the bacon and onions and saute for a couple of minutes. Set aside while leaving a bit of the bacon grease inside the skillet.

- Season the pork chops with salt and pepper and brown on high heat for 3 minutes, then lower the heat and cook for another 3 minutes on each side.
- Return the bacon and onions and finish off with the heavy cream, cooking for another minute.
- Serve ideally with cauliflower rice.

Beef

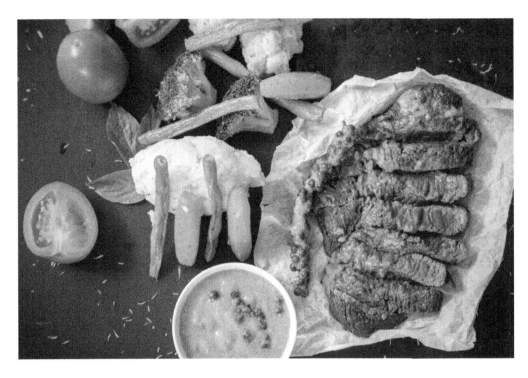

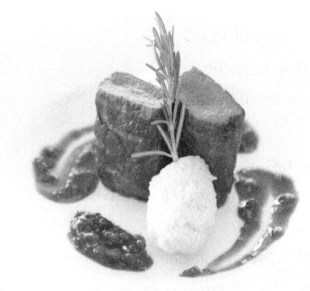

Aromatic Roast Beef

Servings: 5

Cooking time: 50 min

Prep time: 10 min

Nutritional Info (per serving):

Calories: 646

Fat: 27 g

Protein: 93 g

Carbs: 0.1 g

Ingredients:

- 1 lbs of beef sirloin or similar lean cut for roast
- 2 tbsp of mustard
- 2 tbsp of olive oil
- 2 tbsp of garlic salt
- 1 spring of fresh rosemary

Directions:

- Combine the mustard, olive oil, and garlic salt in a small bowl.
- Take the roast beef, remove excess fat and make small incisions lengthwise so you can let the mixture penetrate more easily.

- Brush the mustard mixture over the beef, making sure it all nicely coated.

- Place on a baking dish and arrange the rosemary leaves on the sides, for extra aroma.

- Cook in a preheated oven at 380F/180 C for 50 minutes (for a medium cook inside).

- Serve with mashed sweet potatoes and/or salad.

Beef Filled Zucchini Boats

Servings: 4

Cooking time: 30 min

Prep time: 15 min

Nutritional Info (per serving):

Calories: 280

Fat: 13 g

Protein: 30 g

Carbs; 4.2 g

Ingredients:

- 1 lb of ground beef with around 80% meat and 20% fat ratio
- 1 cup of red Mexican salsa
- 4 medium zucchinis
- ½ shredded cheddar cheese
- 1 tbsp of olive oil

Directions:

- Take the zucchinis, cut in half lengthwise and scoop out the middle flesh inside (leaving enough flesh to make a boat on the sides). Take a form and pinch the insides slightly.

- Heat the pan with the olive oil and add the ground beef.
- Saute for 7-8 minutes or until most of the juices have evaporated.
- Add the salsa and cook for another couple of minutes
- Distribute the ground beef and salsa over the zucchini boats
- Sprinkle with the cheese on top of each.
- Bake in the oven for 15 minutes and serve.

Red Wine Marinated Beef Skewers

Servings: 2-3

Cooking time: 10 min

Prep time: 8-10 min

Nutritional Info (per serving):

Calories: 491

Fat: 24 g

Protein: 55 g

Carbs: 4.8 g

Ingredients:

- 1 lb of sirloin steak cut into cubes
- ½ cup of red dry wine
- 2 tbsp of soy sauce
- 2 tbsp of olive oil
- 8 oz mushrooms

Directions:

- Mix together all the liquids in a bowl to make a marinade
- Take the beef pieces and pass into skewers in this pattern: one beef piece/one mushroom (there will be around 2-3 pieces of each in every skewer)

- Add to the skewered beef and mushrooms to the marinade and let in the fridge for at least an hour before cooking.
- Heat a broiler or grill pan and cook the beef skewers for 3 minutes on each side (for a medium to well-done cook).
- Serve with a green salad.

Chipotle Spicy Steak

Servings: 2

Cooking time: 20 min

Prep time: 5 min

Nutritional Info (per serving):

Calories: 470

Fat: 24 g

Protein: 50 g

Carbs: 4 g

Ingredients:

- 2 sirloin steaks, cut into thin strips
- 1 tbsp of chipotle seasoning powder
- 2 tbsp of olive oil
- ¼ cup tomato paste
- Salt to taste

Directions:

- Combine the tomato paste, olive oil, and chipotle seasoning with salt to make a marinade.
- Brush the mixture onto the steaks.
- Heat a grilling pan and cook the steaks 2-3 minutes on each side for medium inside or depending on how cooked you want them to be.

Cheeseburger Wraps

Servings: 2

Cooking time: 10 min

Prep time: 15 min

Nutritional Info (per serving):

Calories: 456

Fat: 21 g

Protein: 37 g

Carbs: 5 g

Ingredients:

- 8 oz. of ground beef with 20% fat
- ¼ cup chopped onion
- 4 small low carb tortillas
- 2 slices of mild cheddar cheese
- 2 tbsp of salsa

Directions:

- Lightly grease a pan and add the onion and saute for a couple of minutes until almost transparent.
- Add the ground beef and saute for 4-5 minutes or until the juices have evaporated,add the salsa and toss.
- Distribute the ground beef mixture on to the tortilla chips and top with parmesan cheese and serve with a bit of sour cream.

Cheddar Jalapeno Meatloaf

Servings: 5

Cooking time: 35-40 min

Prep time: 5 min

Nutritional Info (per serving):

Calories: 407

Fat: 28.5 g

Protein: 30.77 g

Carbs: 2.3 g

Ingredients:

- 2 lb ground beef
- ½ tsp cumin
- 2 jalapenos, sliced
- 1 1/2 tbsp of garlic salt
- 1 ½ cups of cheddar cheese

Directions:

- Preheat the oven to 375F/180C.
- Combine all the ingredients together except the jalapenos and cheese.

- Fill a deep baking dish (around 8X8 inches) with the ground beef and spice mixture, top with the jalapenos and finish with the layer of cheddar cheese.
- Bake in the oven for 35-40 minutes. Let rest for 5 minutes before serving and cut ideally into squares or triangles before serving.

Grilled Steak and Creamy Mushroom Sauce

Servings: 4

Cooking time: 8 min

Prep time: 5 minutes

Nutritional Info (per serving):

Calories: 636

Fat: 45.68 g

Protein: 7 g

Carbs: 4.3 g

Ingredients:

- 4 New York Strip Steaks
- 10 oz. of a button or regular white mushrooms
- ⅓ cup heavy cream
- 1 tbsp of butter
- Salt/Pepper

Directions:

- Season the steaks on each side with salt and pepper,
- In a shallow skillet, add the butter to melt and then add the mushrooms. Saute for around 3 minutes or until softened.

- Meanwhile, preheat the broiler and add the steaks cooking for 6-7 minutes in total or 3 minutes to each side for a medium-rare result. If you want them more cooked, increase the broiling time a few more minutes.
- Add the heavy cream to the pan with the mushrooms, season with salt and pepper and let heat for 1-2 minutes.
- Pour the mushroom cream sauce over the steaks and serve. This goes well with salad, buttered boiled veggies or cauliflower rice.

Philly Cheesesteak Stuffed Peppers

Servings: 4

Cooking time: 20 min

Prep time: 15 min

Nutritional Info (per serving):

Calories: 458

Fat: 36 g

Protein: 27 g

Carbs: 8 g

Ingredients:

- 2 large bell peppers cut in half lengthwise
- 8 oz. of thinly sliced roast beef or pastrami beef
- 6 oz. of baby mushrooms, sliced
- 8 slices of provolone or cheddar cheese
- 2 tbsp of salted butter

Directions:

- Make sure that the bell peppers are cut lengthwise into halves and contain no seeds.
- In a pan, melt the butter and add the mushrooms. Saute for 3-4 minutes and remove from the heat.
- Take the bell pepper halves and start arranging one slice of cheese over the bottom layer of the pepper,

then 2 slices of pastrami on each and them a few mushrooms. Finish off each pepper boat with an extra slice of cheese on top.

- In a preheated oven (around 400F/200C), pop the peppers and cook for 18-20 minutes so that the peppers are cooked and the cheese is melted.
- Let cool for 5 minutes and serve.

Beef and Eggs Breakfast Muffins

Servings: 12

Cooking time: 15 min

Prep time: 10 min

Nutritional Info (per serving):

Calories: 222

Fat: 18 g

Protein: 15.2 g

Carbs: 1.2 g

Ingredients:

- 2 lbs of ground beef (20% fat/80% lean meat ratio)
- 1 tbsp of mixed herbs
- 12 eggs
- 1 cup of shredded cheddar cheese
- 2 ½ cups of spinach

Directions:

- In a deep pan, saute the spinach with some olive oil for a few minutes until wilted. Remove from the heat and set aside.
- In a 12-piece muffin tin dish begin lining each tin with around 1-2 tbsp of the ground beef to make a

base cup. You should cover all sides of the tin and leave room for the spinach and eggs.

- Top each meat cup with spinach, the cheese and one egg on top.
- Cook in the oven for 15-18 minutes at 400F/200C.

Low Carb Beef Stroganoff

Servings: 7-8

Cooking time: 3 h

Prep time: 15 min

Nutritional Info (per serving):

Calories: 260

Fat: 14. 2 g

Protein: 26 g

Carbs: 6 g

Ingredients:

- 1 lb/500 grams of beef cubes (from steak or sirloin)
- 1 onion, chopped into big pieces
- 1 ½ cup of beef stock
- 3 tbsp of tomato paste
- 1 cup of mushrooms sliced.

Directions:

- Saute optionally the onions and mushrooms with a bit of olive oil and brown the meat only for a couple of minutes.
- Add everything in the slow cooker and cook on high heat for 3 hours.

Vegetarian

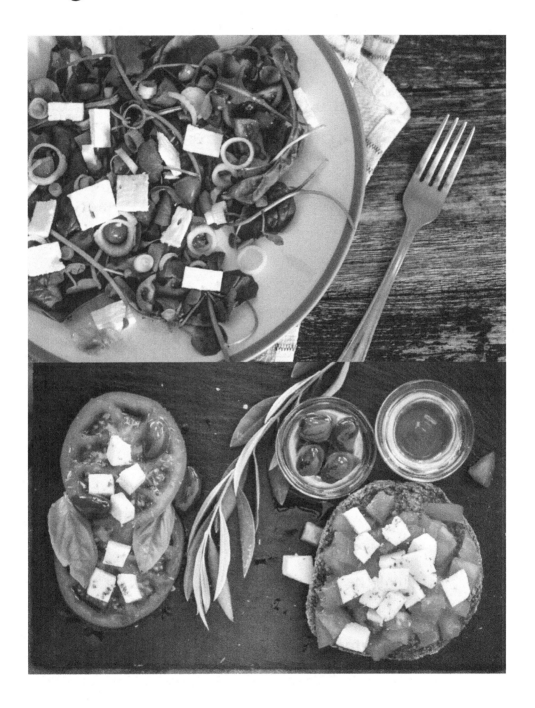

Grilled Halloumi Bruschetta

Servings: 4
Cooking time: 10 min
Prep time: 10 min

Nutritional Info (per serving):

Calories: 134

Fat: 124 g

Protein: 7.24 g

Carbs: 1 g

Ingredients:

- 2 medium tomatoes, chopped
- 2 packages of halloumi cheese (Cyprus grilling cheese), cut into 1 inch thick slices lengthwise
- 2 tbsp of olive oil
- 1 tbsp of chopped fresh basil leaves, chopped

Directions:

- In a bowl combine the tomatoes with the basil and 1 tbsp of the olive oil.
- Heat the remaining tsp of olive oil in a grilling pan and add the halloumi cheese slices to grill, for around 2 minutes on each side.
- Serve the halloumi slices with the tomato mixture on top, as if you are making a bruschetta.

Cheddar Ranch Roasted Cauliflower

Servings: 6

Cooking time: 25-30 min

Prep time: 5 min

Nutritional Info (per serving):

Calories: 81

Fat: 11.68 g

Protein: 2.24 g

Carbs: 3.75 g

Ingredients:

- 1 medium head cauliflower, cut into small 1 in. florets
- 3 tbsp cheddar cheese, shredded (or vegan parmesan cheese)
- ¼ cup ranch dressing
- 3 tbsp of avocado
- Salt/Pepper to taste

Directions:

- Grease a baking dish with the avocado oil
- Arrange the cauliflower florets, season with salt and pepper and toss with the ranch dressing and cheese.
- Bake in the oven for 25 minutes before serving.

Wild Mushroom Soup with Crème Fraiche

Servings: 6

Cooking time: 30 min

Prep time: 10 min

Nutritional Info (per serving):

Calories: 281

Fat: 24.65 g

Protein: 6.11 g

Carbs: 9.12g

Ingredients:

- 10 oz of wild mushrooms
- ¼ cup salted butter
- 1 tbsp of garlic, minced
- 5 cups of vegetable broth
- ½ cup of fresh cream

Directions:

- Heat a pan with the butter and saute the mushrooms with the garlic for 3-4 minutes.
- Transfer to a large saucepan and add the vegetable broth. Bring to a boil and reduce the heat to simmer for 20 minutes.

- Add the creme fresh towards the last two minutes of cooking.

- Let the soup cool for 5 minutes and using an immersion blender blend until the soup is silky smooth with no visible parts of mushrooms. You should end up with a grayish brown sort of color.

- Transfer into soup bowls and add extra doses of cream or parsley on top optionally, for garnish.

Grilled Vegetable Salad with Olive Oil and Feta

Servings: 4

Cooking time: 8 min

Prep time: 10 min

Nutritional Info (per serving):

Calories: 186

Fat: 14 g

Protein: 5 g

Carbs: 12 g

Ingredients:

- 3 grilling vegetables of your choice (e.g eggplant, zucchini, and onions)
- ½ tsp oregano
- ½ cup of crumbled feta
- 2 tbsp of olive oil
- 1 tbsp of balsamic vinegar

Directions:

- In a grilling pan or in the broiler, cut the veggies into slices, season with oregano and salt/pepper and cook until done for around 15 minutes.

- Combine the olive oil and balsamic vinegar in a small cup or bowl to make a vinaigrette.
- Drizzle the vinaigrette over the veggies and top with the crumbled feta pieces and serve.

Low-Carb Pumpkin and Coconut Cream Soup

Servings: 4

Cooking time: 30 min

Prep time: 10 min

Nutritional Info (per serving):

Calories: 234

Fat: 21. 5 g

Protein: 2.3 g

Carbs: 9 g

Ingredients:

- 2 cups of pumpkin chunks
- 2 cups of vegetable stock
- 1 cup of coconut cream
- 1 tbsp of butter
- 1 tsp of ginger powder

Directions:

- Heat a cooking pot and add the butter and the pumpkin chunks. Saute for 3-4 minutes.

- Add the vegetable stock and the ginger powder and bring to a boil. Reduce the heat to simmer for 20-25 minutes.
- Add the coconut cream last and cook for another 2-3 minutes.
- Blend the soup with an immersion blender until creamy smooth. Serve with a drizzle of coconut cream (optionally) on top.

Keto Avocado Pesto Noodles

Servings: 2

Cooking time: 10 min

Prep time: 5 min

Nutritional Info (per serving):

Calories: 321

Fat: 32.7 g

Protein: 0.3 g

Carbs:2 g

Ingredients:

- 1 avocado
- 1 cup of pesto ready-made or homemade pesto sauce
- 1 pack of gluten free or low carb noodles

Directions:

- Cook the noodles as per package instructions.
- Mash the avocado and combine with the pesto sauce.
- Pour over the noodles and toss until well-combined. You can also garnish with red hot peppers on top.

Roasted Radishes with Soy Sauce

Servings: 4

Cooking time: 25 min

Prep time: 5 min

Nutritional Info (per serving):

Calories: 258 g

Fat: 22.7 g

Protein: 5.6 g

Carbs: 9 g

Ingredients:

- 20 small to medium radishes, cut in half
- 2 tbsp of toasted sesame oil
- 1 1/2 tbsp of soy sauce
- 2 green onions, sliced
- 1 tbsp of black sesame seeds

Directions:

- Line a baking tray with parchment paper and place the radishes with 1 tbsp of sesame oil to roast for 20 minutes at 400F/200C.

- Combine the rest of the sesame oil with the soy sauce and the green onions. Add to the roasted radishes and roast everything for another 27-28 minutes.
- Transfer onto a wide dish and sprinkle with some black sesame seeds on top.

Cheesy Vegan Zoodles

Servings: 4

Cooking time: 10 min

Prep time: 5 min

Nutritional Info (per serving):

Calories: 188

Fat: 1.4 g

Protein: 19 g

Carbs: 22 g

Ingredients:

- 4 small zucchinis spiralized into noodles
- ½ cup of diced onion
- ½ cup of red diced pepper
- 3 tbsp of vegetable stock
- ¾ cup nutritional yeast

Directions:

- In a small pot over medium heat, combine the zoodles with the diced pepper and onions and vegetable stock until they have softened and the liquid has evaporated.
- Toss in the nutritional yeast and stir well.
- Serve in 1-2 bowls.

Cauliflower Mac & Cheese

Servings: 6

Cooking time: 45 min

Prep time: 12 min

Nutritional Info (per serving):

Calories: 393

Fat: 33 g

Protein: 14 g

Carbs: 9 g

Ingredients:

- 1 large head of cauliflower, cut into small florets
- 2 ½ cups of shredded cheddar cheese
- 2 cups of full-fat milk
- ¼ cup of salted butter
- Salt/Pepper to taste

Directions:

- Boil the cauliflower florets in boiling salted water for around 10 minutes. Drain and set aside.
- While these are boiling, preheat the oven to 380F/180C.

- Grease a baking tray with the butter and add the cooked cauliflower florets. Season with extra salt and pepper to taste.

- Add the milk, toss and press lightly with a fork to flatten everything up and top with the cheddar cheese.

- Bake for 30 minutes before serving.

Caprese Grilled Eggplant Roll-ups

Servings: 8

Cooking time: 8-10 min

Prep time: 5 min

Nutritional Info (per serving):

Calories: 59

Fat: 3 g

Protein: 3 g

Carbs: 3.8 g

Ingredients:

- 1 eggplant aubergine, cut lengthwise into 7-8 thin slices with a sharp knife.
- 4 oz. of mozzarella
- 1 large tomato, sliced
- A bit of olive oil
- Salt to taste

Directions:

- Season the eggplant slices with salt and drizzle with olive oil.
- In a grilling pan, grill the slices for 3 minutes on each side.

- In a dish or board, arrange one tomato slice over each eggplant slice and top with mozzarella. Roll from left to right and secure with a toothpick.
- Bake in the oven for 10 minutes at 375F/180 C or until cheese is melted.
- Serve.

Drinks and Desserts

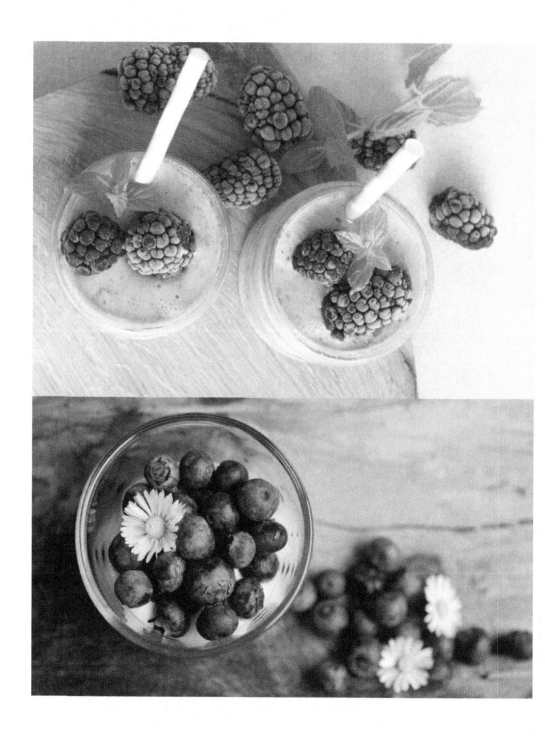

Strawberry Coconut Smoothie

Servings:1

Cooking time: 0

Prep time: 5

Nutritional Info (per serving):

Calories: 128

Fat: 17. 3 g

Protein: 3 g

Carbs: 9.2 g

Ingredients:

- 5 frozen strawberries
- 1 ½ cup of unsweetened coconut milk
- 1 tbsp of vanilla flavored Greek yogurt

Directions:

- Combine everything in a blender until smooth.
- Transfer to a glass or mason jars and enjoy chilled.

Keto Avocado Ice Cream

Servings: 6

Cooking time:1 h

Prep time: 12 min

Nutritional Info (per serving):

Calories: 255

Fat: 92 g

Protein: 7 g

Carbs: 12 g

Ingredients:

- 2 big ripe avocados
- 1 can of full fat and unsweetened coconut milk
- 2 tbsp of stevia or honey
- 1 tbsp of lime juice

Directions:

- Blend everything together in a blender until you end up with a creamy smooth consistency.
- Transfer the mixture onto an ice cream maker or popsicle molds (if you don't have an ice cream maker) and freeze for at least an hour before serving.

Ketto Chai Latte

Servings: 2

Cooking time: 5 min

Prep time: 1 min

Nutritional Info (per serving):

Calories: 135

Fat: 14 g

Protein: 1 g

Carbs: 1 g

Ingredients:

- 1 chai tea bag
- 2 cups of water
- ½ whipping cream
- ½ tsp of cinnamon powder

Directions:

- Brew the chai tea bag in hot water for 5 minutes.
- Transfer into two small cups and add some whipping cream on top.
- Sprinkle a bit of cinnamon powder.

Sugar-free Lemon Curd

Servings: 1 cup

Cooking time: 10 min

Prep time: 10 min

Nutritional Info (per serving):

Calories: 258

Fat: 25 g

Protein: 7 g

Carbs: 2 g

Ingredients:

- 4 unwaxed lemons (juice and zest kept)
- ⅓ cup of erythritol or stevia
- 100 grams of unsalted butter
- 3 whole eggs
- 1 egg yolk

Directions:

- Get a medium bowl and squeeze out the lemons and zest half of their skin.
- Add the stevia or erythritol and the butter.

- Heat a pan with boiling water and add the bowl with the lemon mixture on toe (ben-Marie method). Careful so that the water doesn't touch the bowl.
- Stir the mixture until the butter has melted.
- Reduce to low heat and carefully whisk in the eggs. Keep stirring constantly and cook for 10 minutes. You should end up with a thin conditioner-like texture.
- Remove from the heat and place on a sterilized jar or jars.

Keto Peanut Butter Cookies

Servings: 15

Cooking time: 12 min

Prep time: 5 min

Nutritional Info (per serving):

Calories: 108

Fat: 9.2 g

Protein: 4.2 g

Carbs: 4.7 g

Ingredients:

- 1 large egg
- 1 cup of unsalted peanut butter or almond butter
- ½ cup of stevia

Directions:

- Preheat the oven at 350F/175C.
- Combine everything together until you end up with a dough-like mixture.
- Make around 15 small balls and press with your hand lightly to flatten.
- Transfer to a baking tray lined with parchment paper or some cookie forms.
- Cook for around 15 minutes.

Conclusion

Following a keto diet couldn't be easier with these (up to) 5 ingredient recipes. They are so easy, filling and delicious that you won't miss the carbs. For the sake of better meal prep and falling within a decent calorie and macronutrient limit to facilitate weight loss, I have included a sample meal plan that will work for the average person. Feel free thought to adjust it according to your tastes and nutritional needs.

Even though Keto diet isn't 100% for everyone, those who wish to lose weight, lower their cholesterol levels, and enjoy a vast array of health benefits will find the diet totally useful and easy to follow.

When following a Keto diet for weight loss, it would also be wise to both count your macro intake level and then your calories so you can get the results you want. In general, a 1500 calorie intake is suggested for most cases, but there is also a basic formula to find out exactly how many calories you should consume when on Keto to lose a decent amount of weight per week or month. Here is how to figure it out:

Energy stored = Energy in - Energy out.

Example: Let's suppose that your body needs 1800 calories to carry out its daily tasks and you only consume 1300 calories. The rest 500 calories will be taken by your body by your stored fat deposits and therefore, you'll lose fat (around 1 lbs of fat in this case).

Keep in mind that the above is a basic formula and the exact amount of daily calories varies from person to person. If you are a busy person with a hectic schedule, for example, you will need to consume more calories to keep yourself energized as you will burn off more calories with each task as opposed to a person that sits and stays inactive or sleeps for the most part.

If you aren't a person on the go, it is also suggested that you do some mild exercising or any mild physical activity that helps you burn more calories without exhausting yourself. Done right and you could lose up 2 lbs per week...

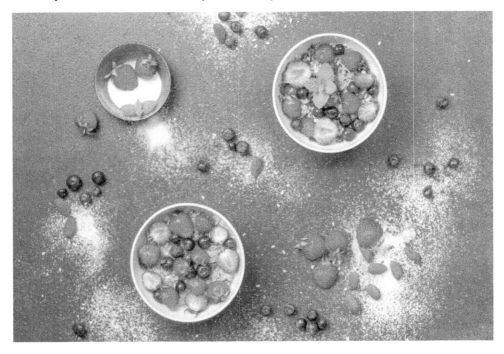

Bonus 14-day Meal Plan

Week 1:

	MON	TUE	WED	THU	FRI	SAT	SUN
Break-fast	Straw-berry Coconut Smoothie	1 hard boiled egg	Ketto Chai Latte	Chicken Club Lettuce Wraps	Spicy avocado filled tuna bowls.	Pizza Pork Rinds	Scotch eggs
Lunch	Creamy Marsala Pork	Turkey meat-balls and zoodles	Cheese Stuffed Pork Meatballs	Easy Bacon Wrapped pork loin	Baked Salmon with Pesto	Low Carb Asian Spareribs	Beef Stroganoff
Snack / Dessert	Grilled Halloumi Bruschetta		2 scoops of avocado ice cream		5 Keto Peanut Butter Cookies		1 tbsp of lemon curd
Dinner	Sausage, shrimp, and zucchini skewers	Roasted Radishes with Soy Sauce	Cheesy Vegan Zoodles	Beef-filled zucchini boats	Low carb-pumpkin and coconut soup	Wild Mushroom soup with creme fraiche	Cheddar Roasted Ranch Cauliflower

134

Week 2:

	MON	TUE	WED	THU	FRI	SAT	SUN
Break-fast	Beef & Eggs breakfast muffins	Grilled Halloumi Bruschetta	4-5 sausage rolls	Coconut strawberry smoothie	Ketto Chai Latte	Spicy avocado filled tuna bowls	1 fried egg and one bacon
Lunch	Asian Glazed Salmon and	Easy spicy pork chops	Crispy Chicken tenders	Red Wine Marinated Beef Skewers	Bacon and onion smothered pork chops	Easy Indian Tikka Masala chicken	Tarragon roasted chicken
Snack / Dessert	Keto peanut butter cookies	1 tbsp of lemon curd on gluten-free bread	5-6 carrot sticks and ranch dressing	Turkey breast nachos	1 orange, sliced	2 scoops of keto ice-cream	1 pear
Dinner	Philly cheese steak stuffed peppers	Grilled steak and mushroom sauce	Baked Lobster tails with garlic butter	Grilled vegetable salad with feta	Keto Avocado Pesto Noodles	Prosciutto wrapped scallops and spinach	Cauliflower mac and cheese

***

Cheers to your Keto Diet Success!

Made in the USA
Columbia, SC
28 March 2021